Weight Loss Solutions Your Body Will Accept

Frederick Mickel Huck

Bloomington, IN 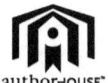 Milton Keynes, UK

authorHOUSE™

AuthorHouse™
1663 Liberty Drive, Suite 200
Bloomington, IN 47403
www.authorhouse.com
Phone: 1-800-839-8640

AuthorHouse™ UK Ltd.
500 Avebury Boulevard
Central Milton Keynes, MK9 2BE
www.authorhouse.co.uk
Phone: 08001974150

First published by AuthorHouse   7/13/2006

ISBN: 1-4259-4346-2 (sc)

Library of Congress Control Number: 2006905305

Printed in the United States of America
Bloomington, Indiana

This book is printed on acid-free paper.

This Book is Dedicated to

ROBERT E. MENZIE

INEZ A. MENZIE

DONALD WALTER HUCK

DOCTOR EDE KOENIG

And Special Thanks to

SANDRA MOONEY

MATTHEW MOONEY

PARVIN MALEK

TARA SHABAFROOZ

ANGIE INGERSOLL

Notes from the Author

Today, I have a higher quality of life, where I continue to help anyone who wants to make this change. I start with food samples, such as desserts, because most people think healthy eating excludes sweets in their diet. I have numerous recipes for desserts including cookies, cakes, pies, ice cream, candy bars, and even fudge.

I talk about the physical condition that I was in before I made this major change in my lifestyle. I had blackouts due to diabetes, where my sugar levels were high; there was blood in my urine, due to diagnosed kidney stones. The kidney stones also caused backaches with various degrees of back pain. I had loose teeth and other bone problems, and I was also fifty-five pounds overweight. Changing my way of life made a major impact on my health-related problems without any surgery or the use of any medication.

Now I am going to share with you how easily this can be done by eating healthily and having colon cleansings. They helped in ridding the body of toxins, worms, bacteria, and parasites.

I feel so much better, with more energy, strength, and thought power. I know that I am not limited anymore, and I am not going back to being sick or to eating junk foods. I will share with you my true story of eating junk food and working out at a gym. For five years, I attended aerobic classes for approximately 250 hours a year, including running around 800 miles each year. I weighed the same for most of the five years with no change. Now I am healthy with fewer daily workouts, maintaining my weight, feeling better, and I enjoy what I eat. If you go to a gym, my recommendation is yoga and walking on the treadmill in an inclined position, keeping the stomach in and the butt muscle tight. Utilizing the dry sauna is also beneficial for the entire body, which is good for the circulation, surface toxins, and it increases blood to the heart. If you do not go to the gym, I recommend a "Cellerciser™" (see back of book) which utilizes the body's gravity; this is a perfect workout.

The biggest inspiration to author this book was not due to a college education —there was no interest or ability to even commit to expensive research — instead it was a healthy body and the desire to help others.

Contents

Introduction

If you are interested in permanent weight loss without the use of drugs and starvation, I have the information you need. Understanding the cause of being overweight is equally as important as losing the weight. The reason why people are having weight problems is the advice they are receiving is only a temporary fix, not an actual solution. I say quit listening to anyone who says it is ok to be unhealthy. Numerous publications, television advertisements, surgical procedures, and companies focused on weight loss continue to drown us with promises of becoming healthy and slimmer. Simple observation reveals obesity as still being a major problem in our society. Life long results can be achieved using common sense; it does not take a PhD! The cause is in two parts: anything put into the body and anything put on the body.

What should be put into the body? Real and whole foods, such as: nuts, grains, fruits, and vegetables. With these four food groups, not only does the body get what it wants, but it also gets everything it needs nutritionally. With these four food groups, you can make anything you are currently eating, with the exception of animal products.

What the body does not want!

Any animal products, over processed sugar, table salt, chemicals, free oils, saturated and unsaturated oils, and overly-processed foods — all of the above equals malnutrition. (Which means lack of nutrition?) This means the body is not getting what it needs. If this continues, the body will malfunction. This is the cause of weight gain.

What should not go on the body?

Stop all Aluminum products, chemicals, animal products, fluoride, artificial colors, and imitation ingredients that are all toxins that the body does not want.

Diets of the past and some new ones

When the body does not get enough nutrition, you will eat more and more junk food, and will continue to be hungry. None of the diets address the cause of the extra weight; common sense should tell you that it is not working. Looking at the popular diets and the history like taking drugs, cutting down on junk foods, eating in moderation, eating six meals a day, increasing exercise, consuming diet drinks, nutrition in a can, nutrition bars, and the list goes on and on. Counting calories does not work; if you are counting calories, you are eating overly processed foods. All this talk equals starvation and hunger pains, and will not work. Some people can lose weight temporarily, but it is still unhealthy.

If you continue to work against the body's immune system, you will lose out against your immune system and your body will continue to malfunction. Listen! How is your body supposed to work properly if you are not treating it with proper nutrition? So, in other words, the weight lost will be back on the body and more.

I used to be in the same situation and looking for another diet to try, and more time and dollars were spent, and the results were the same. Remember that you cannot work against your body. By remembering the reasons why the last diet did not work should be very simple because malnutrition never works.

I do believe everyone has a choice. Do you want to continue to be overweight or do you not want to be overweight? That is your choice. The problem of being overweight is to stop abusing your body. Make the changes needed to solve this problem.

If you make some changes, you will see some results within fourteen days, but I do caution you: Why do you want to make only some changes? Your body expects more. The more you treat your body with proper nutrition, the more weight loss will occur.

My plan will include basic cooking and basic nutrition, and is designed for the beginner. I promise it will be very rewarding, inexpensive, and save you time. All of the food can be made to your taste, and the recipes are in large print and easy to read and follow. The food is delicious and I found that there is more variety. I always say to new people, I am no longer restricted like I used to be in the past. There is no comparison in the junk food and what I have today. I believe there is more garbage in fast food, which I used to eat, than I ever imagined.

I recommend two meals a day, morning and afternoon. The meals should be eaten five hours apart from each other, from beginning to end. Let us say you started eating at 6:30 AM and ended at 7:00 AM. Wait at least five hours or more, then you can eat your second meal. As for water, no water is drunk during a meal. Half an hour before a meal is ok. Drink all the water you want two hours after a meal. Ice cold water is good at night to curb your appetite if you feel a little hungry.

Food Preparation

Most meals are simple to prepare and very basic, and some take more labor to prepare. That is why the recipes are designed to cook in bulk. If you do this, it will give you more free time. Based on my experience I have saved up to 80 percent savings on my food bill. All this food is delicious and saves you time.

What about sweets? My response is: Which ones? I have several recipes (see back of book) for cakes, pies, cookies, ice cream, and candy.

I have recipes for everything I used to eat, but the difference is, it is not junk food. This is food for the body. I believe that if I can duplicate the foods that I used to enjoy, why go back to junk foods? My sweets taste so much better and I am not limited like I used to be. I am not sick anymore and I have more of a social life. Now that I look back to when I used to eat in restaurants, I never could eat and talk at the same time.

When do you want to eat the best? When do you want to eat delicious food? When will you be ready? Later on, I will include some cooking tips and how to set up your own pantry, step by step, with easy-to-follow recipes. You will enjoy these tasty meals. Don't you deserve it?

For Thanksgiving, I made dinner for ten adults, who were enjoying a healthy meal which included a holiday roast, the size of a cookie tray. The dinner also included a large cookie-tray-sized cornbread, twelve yams with pineapple sauce, and two pumpkin pies with whipped cream. All this cost only thirty-four dollars, and everyone stayed full until breakfast. Since this was a special to-go order, this did not include if any of the adults had vegetables or a salad.

Setting up the pantry

*(SOME ITEMS WILL HAVE TO BE REFRIGERATED
OR PLACED IN A FREEZER AFTER OPENING)*

Popcorn - it should be dry popcorn

Braggs amino - a natural soy sauce – it must be refrigerated after opening. Example-can be used for salads, beans, rice or pasta

Coconut Lite 8.8 ounces powder – a fine powder used for cooking

Tofu – (I recommend Mori-Nu Tofu) ingredients: water, soybeans, gluconlastone, and calcium chloride

Sage, celery seeds, dill weed, ground marjoram, turmeric, whole caraway seeds

Soy milk – ingredients: organic whole soybeans, rice syrup, filtered water, sea salt

Vitamix – or a blender

Pure vanilla – no alcohol

Puffed rice – puffed corn

Maple Syrup – 100%

Roma coffee – (ingredients: roasted malt, barley, roasted barley, roasted chicory)

Carob- chocolate substitute

Tapioca – for thickening; grind into a fine powder

Corn tortillas – brand name Mi Rancho; ingredients: water, corn, and lime

Canned green olives – ingredients: olives, water, and salt

Tomato paste –tomato only (no salt), can be bought in a can

Cereals – stay away from any sugar, any oil, and any fructose; look for whole grains only

Oatmeal – old fashioned Quaker oats, 100% whole grain and natural only

Ezekiel bread – 4:9 brand, they make a sesame seed wheat, cinnamon, rye bread.

Organic Sucanat Sugar-natural certified sweetener (brown colored only). The brand is Natural Touch: Wholesome Sweetener

Teflon cooking trays – stainless steel pots and pans, or glass

Cookie mats – parchment paper

Pasta - 100% durum wheat semolina – ingredients: niacin, ferrous lactate, (iron) thiamin, Mononitrate, riboflavin, and folic acid

Oregano, ground thyme

Corn – fresh or frozen (no salt)

Peas – fresh or frozen (no salt)

Pineapple – fresh or in a can – ingredients: 100% pineapple, pineapple juice, water, and Certified pineapple juice concentrate

Bio-salt

Inland sea water

Lemons – fresh

Whole cornmeal

Corn flour

Apricot pits (Is Vit B-17) – the nut inside the pit, raw / best to buy in Middle Eastern market

Brazil nuts – raw

Pumpkin seeds – raw

Paprika

Garlic powder

Almonds – raw

Sunflower seeds – raw

Parsley flakes

Red chilies – fresh or dry flakes

Whole caraway seeds

Celery seeds

Ground ginger

Chili powder

Cayenne pepper

Italian seasonings

Cinnamon – ground

Cumin

Onion – dried

Dry yeast – is only used to make dough rise

Whole summer savory leaf

Pristine oil – is used instead of toothpaste, because toothpaste is composed of sand, fluoride, and other chemicals

Herbal Magnesium: (must have kelp) rue, black walnut – whole, black walnut leaf, butcher's broom, oat straw.

Herbal Calcium, horsetail, comfrey, dandelion root, alfalfa, oat straw, parsley root, and lobelia; these ingredients are all natural and based on herbs.

The calcium and magnesium supplements that arc typically available are not based on herbs but rather chemical and or animals base, that the body will reject. Dr. Ede Koenig, has formulated an herbal form of calcium and magnesium where one-eighth of a teaspoon equals one capsule. Two capsules of each supplement are taken with each meal.

The Restaurant Test

Any restaurants using any of the following stay away! White flour, polished white rice, over processed sugar, table salt, MSG, any oil, any chemicals, any animal products, canned fruits and vegetables, mushrooms, bananas, black pepper, any kind of vinegar, natural flavors, artificial flavors and colors.

Unsanitary restaurants, even with the best intentions in mind, have some unsanitary conditions. Some may be slight and others may be unacceptable. As much cooking as I do, I can understand how easily these conditions can exist; however, I do practice sanitary cooking.

Fast Food Restaurants

Fast food is not fast. Just add up the time it takes to drive to and from any establishment and add the time you wait in line. I can make any food quicker than a fast food establishment. My food is 80 percent lower in cost than any restaurant. I will never eat in any restaurant, not even if it is free. I will not limit myself to what I eat by going into a restaurant.

The Dos and Don'ts

The don'ts: vinegar, unsaturated oils, saturated oils, bananas, (they lack nutrition due to being picked too green), mushrooms (are a *fungus*), peanuts (are loaded with *Aflotoxins*), iceberg lettuce (has Opium), any beans in a can (high in sodium), tomato on a salad (the tomato equals a fruit unless you boil it for two hours), fruits and veggies (do not mix together), any aluminum products; black and green tea are high in caffeine, Tannic Acid, table salt (there is fructose in salt, which is over processed sugar), black pepper, chocolate, and Theo Broimine are high in caffeine, insect parts and rat hairs.

The dos: only one quarter pound a day of desserts. One half avocado, one teaspoon sunflower seeds, eight brazil nuts (raw) — they are high in selenium — one teaspoon of raw pumpkin seeds, six apricot seeds, two raw almonds daily, herbal calcium, herbal magnesium, ozone technology, hydrogen peroxide, yeast (if using yeast to make anything rise, after it is cooked, let cool down and put in the refrigerator for three days, then you can eat it, because the yeast enzymes will be dead by then).

Hydrogen peroxide: When cleaning fruits and vegetables, use one-quarter of a cup of hydrogen peroxide in a sink of water, and then weigh down with a dish. Keep it there for half an hour; you can do this several times. Mix to get dirt and debris off; hydrogen peroxide will kill parasites.

The Diet Test

Instead of listing all the diets of the past and present, I have a diet test. If your diet includes or promotes any of the following, do not waste your time or money. It will not work in the long term and you will still be unhealthy: drugs, body alterations, eating several small meals daily, diets in a can, diets in an energy bar, diet drinks, counting calories, cutting down on what you are presently eating, any animal products, products containing caffeine, products containing chocolate, and imitation food. All I am saying is that these diets equal starvation due to the lack of nutrition and they all work with the symptoms instead of the cause. That is why they do not work.

Colon Hydro Therapy (or colon cleanse)

After your eating problems have been established, I recommend colonics. It may take a few days for the body to adjust, and then I recommend that you do colonics. Six one-hour sessions, one every day, will clean the large and small intestines and other parts of the body. I even witnessed stones coming out of the body. This process also removes worms, parasites, bacteria, and toxins from the body that do not belong there. When you are eating healthy you will not be putting then back in there.

A colon therapist should be consulted for this procedure. If you cannot find one, contact a doctor of nutrition, and they can find one for you. Do not be part of a system that does not work! Just look at the results of the many doctors who say it is ok to eat junk food, as long as it is eaten only in moderation. Only real foods should be eaten; you are in charge of your body. You manage it, not someone who has an interest in your being sick. It does not take a college degree to figure this out; mistreating your body does not make sense. Do not continue to do this. My plan is here if you want it to work for you. You should see incrediable results in two weeks.

Hand Nut Grinder

Do not use the hand nut grinder for hazelnuts, almonds, or Brazil nuts. You could damage the grinder blade. I did this, and my friend Gus found in his hazelnut fudge a piece of metal the size of one-third of a toothpick. Luckily there was no damage to his teeth or gums, because he was chewing slowly. Instead, use a long knife to chop nuts or place them in a heavy plastic bag and crush them with a rolling pin. The hand grinder is for walnuts and pecans only.

Breads

I use tonir lavash, 100 percent wheat flour, yeast, salt, and water.

Nutritional facts: Sodium is 105 mg, 4%. You can find this bread in a delicatessen; you must find out when the bread is made. My bread is delivered the same day it is baked, which is Tuesday, so Friday I can eat this bread. The yeast dissipates when you put it in warm water, however the volatile gas does not dissipate for three days.

Recipes

Recipe 1 _____

Baked Potato

In a brown bag, place two to four clean potatoes in a microwave oven. Start with five minutes; to see if the potato is cooked, test with a fork. If the fork goes into the potato easily, it is cooked. The cooking time may vary because of the differences in microwaves. I put a little lemon juice and Braggs-amino on them.

Recipe 2 _____

Salads

I recommend red leaf, green leaf, or romaine lettuce. One stalk of celery, one third of a carrot, three radishes (red), cilantro to your taste, one half of an avocado, one long green onion, six teaspoons of fresh lemon juice, six to twelve ounces of two different hot sauces, one teaspoon of Braggs-amino or more.

Recipe 3 ———————————————

Pasta

Follow the boiling instructions on the bag, because different shapes and sizes of pasta vary. You can use any kind of pasta, as long as it is 100 percent Durum wheat. Usually, I boil one pound of pasta for ten minutes. Pour out the water and pasta into a strainer and pour an additional half gallon of fresh water on the pasta — this will keep the pasta from sticking.

Recipe 4 ———————————————

Pasta sauce — tomato sauce

This recipe is called tomato sauce and requires 22 tomatoes, or 22 cups of tomatoes placed in a blender with eight cups of water. Then pour it into a large pan with the following: four cloves of garlic cut small, two bell peppers cut small, two teaspoons of basil, two teaspoons of dill, two tablespoons bio – salt, two teaspoons of cumin, and one can of green olives cut small, four teaspoons of Italian seasoning, one onion cut small, one shredded carrot, one stalk of celery cut small, and one tablespoon maple syrup. Bring to a boil, and then turn to low for two hours. Add to top of pasta, as much as desired; if desired, add cayenne pepper to taste.

Recipe 5 ———————————————

Brown Rice

In a pan, soak rice overnight. Use six cups of rice with eight cups of water; add one tablespoon of bio-salt and stir. For cooking the next day, bring to a boil, place lid on pan, then turn to low heat. The rice should be cooked within fifteen minutes. Check to see if all the water is gone in the pan.

Recipe 6

Texan Rice

In a pan, add two teaspoons of Braggs-amino, one teaspoon of bio-salt, half of a bell pepper — red, green, orange, or yellow does not matter — half of an onion (chopped), one tablespoon of chili powder, six tomatoes cut small, and two cups of whole corn. Boil for fifteen minutes or more on low heat; most of the liquid should be gone. Stir and place six ounces of cooked lentils, six ounces of cooked pinto beans. Add this to the cooked rice. See recipe #5. Remember to add all of these into the same pan of cooked rice, stir mixture, and turn off the heat. Place lid on pan and let sit until pan is cooled. Freeze extra in six-ounce cup until needed.

Recipe 7

Bell pepper rice

In a pan, add the following:

One bell pepper, cut small (red, orange, or yellow)

One onion, cut small

One can of green olives, cut up in halves

One half cup of cilantro, cut small

Four teaspoons of Braggs-amino

Two tablespoons of parsley

One teaspoon of garlic powder

One teaspoon of paprika

Three tablespoons of lemon juice

One teaspoon of bio-salt

Boil on low heat for fifteen minutes or more and stir frequently; the liquid should be mostly gone, and then add to the cooked rice. See recipe #5. Stir so the mixture is mixed into the rice. Turn off the heat, place the lid on the pan, and let sit until cooled.

Recipe 8 ⎯⎯⎯⎯⎯⎯⎯⎯⎯⎯⎯⎯⎯⎯⎯⎯⎯⎯⎯⎯⎯⎯

Tostadas

Toast corn tortillas or wheat tortillas, let cool down and add beans to the shell, then add salad mixture. The mixture is:

One green long onion, chopped small

Three radishes cut small

Half of an avocado

Add to taste on top of this: lemon juice, hot sauce, Braggs-amino.

See bean recipe #11

Recipe 9 ⎯⎯⎯⎯⎯⎯⎯⎯⎯⎯⎯⎯⎯⎯⎯⎯⎯⎯⎯⎯⎯⎯

Popcorn

Use only dry popcorn, and place into a brown bag, pop into a microwave oven, then let cool. You can add Braggs-amino spray.

Recipe 10 _____

Hot sauce

Place in a blender:

21 tomatoes or 21 cups of tomatoes

Four cloves of garlic

One cup of red crushed peppers (optional)

Two tablespoons of dill

One tablespoon of bio-salt

Four tablespoons of cumin

One half cup of maple syrup

Half a cup of cilantro

Bring to a boil on high heat and turn to low for two hours; you can freeze the extra until needed.

Recipe 11 _____

Cindy Huck Beans for Burritos

The night before, soak five cups of beans — pinto, red, black, etc, except lentils; in a pan with water one to two inches above the beans. The next day, boil on high for ten minutes, then pour out the water and replace that water with water one to two inches above the beans. Then add one tablespoon of bio-salt, one clean potato with skin to soak up volatile substance that beans have. After the beans are cooked, throw away the potato. Let boil on high, then switch to low heat until cooked. Cooking time: approximately 30-40 minutes.

Recipe 12 _____

Todd Neumiller Chinese soup

Boil one gallon of water and add one half cup of the following:

Thin pasta noodles

Cooked rice (brown)

Lentils (cooked)

Cabbage

Celery

Carrots (cut small or shredded)

Lemon juice

One tablespoon of paprika

One cup of Braggs-amino

One half teaspoon of marjoram

One half teaspoon of maple syrup

Boil on low for one hour; you can freeze the extra.

Recipe 13 _____

Almond butter

Roast three pounds of raw almonds in the oven on a cookie sheet for 30 minutes at 325 degrees. Let cool one to two hours, and then grind in the Vitamix on high until the butter is very smooth.

Place in a bowl and then add one half teaspoon of bio-salt and continue to mix; the extra can be frozen if placed in jars.

Recipe 14 ────────────────────

Pizza sauce

Start by placing 18 tomatoes or 18 cups of tomatoes into a blender. Add six cups of water only. Depending on the size of your blender, you may need to grind only six tomatoes and two cups of water at a time.

Then pour into a large pan with the following:

One chopped onion

One can of green olives (each olive cut in half)

Four cloves of garlic cut small

One bell pepper cut small

Two teaspoons of cumin

Two teaspoons of oregano

Four teaspoons of paprika

One teaspoon of marjoram

Three teaspoons of maple syrup

Boil for two hours on low heat. The sauce must be thick like paste. Apply to cooked pizza dough before serving; you can freeze the extra into twelve-ounce cups.

Recipe 15 _____

Pizza dough (for pie)

In a bowl, mix one teaspoon of almond butter

One quarter teaspoon of bio-salt

One half cup of warm water; you can add a little more afterwards

Then stir in one and half cups of whole-wheat pastry flour, sifted, and add one tablespoon of yeast. Mix with clean hands. Knead the dough; it could take five minutes. The dough should not be sticky, and if it is sticky, it means that you have used too much water. If the dough is too dry, you can add more water, one teaspoon at a time; roll into a ball, and form into a pie crust. Line a 9 x 9-inch round pan with parchment paper, press dough into the pan. You can add poppy seeds, cornmeal, and sesame seeds, pressed into the dough.

Bake at 425 degrees for ten to thirteen minutes. Dough should be soft. Just before eating, pour twelve ounces or less of pizza sauce into a pie; place back into 250-degree oven for fifteen to twenty minutes, <u>just before eating.</u>

Recipe 16 _____

Waffles

You can use any waffle iron. In a blender, add the following:

Two and a half cups of water

One and a half cups of rolled plain oats

One third cup of raw almonds

One quarter cup of sunflower seeds (raw)

One half teaspoon of bio-salt

Add batter into the waffle iron; bake twelve to fifteen minutes, depending on how crispy you want it. You can freeze the extra.

Recipe 17

Tamale casserole

<u>First,</u> boil the following for fifteen minutes:

Four cups of whole corn

One bell pepper, cut small

One onion, cut small

One can of green olives, each cut in half

Two tomatoes cut small

Three tablespoons of Braggs-amino

Boil until most of the juice is gone. Set it aside.

<u>Second,</u> put the following in a blender:

Three tablespoons of garlic powder

Two tablespoons of onion powder

One tablespoon of maple syrup

Four cups of soy milk

One tablespoon of chili powder

Four teaspoons of cumin

Four teaspoons of bio-salt

Six tomatoes

<u>Third,</u> pour everything into a large bowl with four cups of cornmeal, and two cups of whole-wheat pastry flour, sifted. Line a 13 x 9 glass dish with parchment paper. Bake at 350 degrees for one hour.

Recipe 18 ——————————

Maple Syrup Cake

Add and mix in a large bowl

2 tablespoon almond butter

1 tablespoon bio-salt

1 tablespoon vanilla

6 cups maple syrup

2 tablespoon rose water

6 cups ground walnuts

4 cups sifted whole-wheat pasty flour

Pour all the ingredients into a 13 x 9-inch baking dish lined with parchment paper.

Bake in a 350-degree oven for approximately 50 minutes. Check to see if baked; use a toothpick to see if center is cooked. If toothpick comes out without extra batter, cake is baked. If toothpick has batter, then continue baking and check every five minutes.

Recipe 19 —————————————————————

Pan-fried noodles

I recommend <u>Udon</u> – Japanese macaroni products; the ingredients:

Wheat flour and sea salt

First boil five quarts of water for ten minutes in a large pan, and add the following:

One half cup of cabbage

One half cup of long green onions, chopped

One half cup of celery, cut small

One half cup of carrots, shredded

One half cup of radishes, cut small

Then add 8.8 ounces of noodles. Continue to boil eight to ten minutes; see the package instructions. After they are cooked, drain in strainer, and let cool and divide into six-ounce cups. You can freeze the extra.

Recipe 20 —————————————————————

Fruit icing

In a blender, place the following:

One half cup of any fresh fruit

Two cups of sucanat sugar

Three tablespoons of soy milk

This can be added to cakes or toast.

Recipe 21 ───────────────────────

Carob baked Alaska

In a blender place the following:

One brick of tofu, or one pound

One cup of maple syrup

One cup of almond butter

One quarter cup of carob powder

One quarter cup of Roma

One half cup sucanat sugar

Mix and place this in seven-inch baking cups. Place these cups in an oven and bake for twenty minutes at 350 degrees. I use the same baking cups for my pot pies.

Recipe 22 ───────────────────────

Vanilla cake

Mix in a blender the following:

One half cup of tofu

One half teaspoon of bio-salt

One tablespoon of almond butter

Half a cup of sucanat sugar

One teaspoon of vanilla

Half cup of soy milk

Then pour the above into a bowl with one and a half cups of whole-wheat pastry flour, sifted with one tablespoon of yeast. Pour all the ingredients into a 9 x 9-inch pan lined with parchment paper (a round pan).

If making two layer cakes, double the recipe; bake at 325 degrees for 45-50 minutes. See recipe #18 for toothpick test.

Recipe 23 ——————————————————————

Carob glaze

By hand, mix in a bowl:

Two cups of sucanat sugar

One quarter cup of carob powder

Three tablespoons of soy milk

Two tablespoons of maple syrup

If it is too thick, you can add one tablespoon of soy milk until thinner. If this is for a cake, double the recipes, let cake cool, and apply.

Recipe 24 ——————————————————————

Maple oatmeal cookies

In a large bowl, add and mix by hand the following:

Eight tablespoons of almond butter

Two teaspoons of vanilla

Two teaspoons of bio-salt

Six cups of maple syrup

Eight cups of oatmeal flour (Oatmeal flour is oatmeal ground in a blender, four cups at a time.) You can let sit for two or three hours if batter is too thin. Form cookies on a cookie sheet lined with parchment paper or you may line with a cookie mat. Bake at 325 degrees for twenty minutes.

Recipe 25 _____

Clove cookies

Mix by hand the following in a large bowl:

One half cup of almond butter

One half teaspoon of cloves, powdered

One teaspoon of vanilla

One quarter cup of tofu

One half cup of maple syrup

One half cup of sucanat sugar

One cup of whole-wheat pastry flour, sifted (can let batter sit for 2 hours)

Bake in oven at 375 degrees for fifteen minutes, after lining cookie sheet with parchment paper or baking mat.

Recipe 26 _____

Donald W. Huck coconut cookies

Mix in a large bowl the following:

Two cups of oatmeal flour (see recipe #24)

Six cups of maple syrup

One teaspoon of bio-salt

Two teaspoons of almond butter

Four cups of raw coconut

Five cups of whole-wheat pastry flour

Mix again, line cookie sheets with parchment paper or baking mat

Bake in the oven for 25 minutes at 325 degrees

Recipe 27 ———————————

Carob Roma Oatmeal Cookies

In a large bowl, mix the following:

Eight teaspoons of almond butter

Six cups of maple syrup

Two teaspoons of vanilla

Two teaspoons of bio-salt

One half cup of Roma

One half cup of carob

Eight cups of oatmeal flour

Stir and add:

Four cups of whole-wheat pastry flour, sifted

You can let it stand for two to three hours because dough is very thin. Place on cookie mat or tray lined with parchment paper. Form into cookie size. Bake in 325-degree oven for 20 minutes. Oatmeal flour is made by putting 100% whole oats in a blender.

Recipe 28 _____

Deep-Dish Pizza

Place in a large bowl and mix the following:

Two cups of sifted whole-wheat pastry flour

One half teaspoon of bio-salt

Two teaspoons of almond butter

Two-thirds cup of lukewarm water

Add one tablespoon of yeast. Mix by hand. The dough must be elastic and knead two or three more minutes. Place in a bowl and put in a warm area. Cover until dough has doubled in size, approximately fifteen to twenty minutes. Knead the dough again for two to three minutes. Form into a circle.

Place in a 9 x 9-inch pan, lined with parchment paper. Bake at 425 degrees for ten minutes. For dinner, add twelve ounces of pizza sauce. Re-bake at 250 degrees for fifteen minutes or until warm whenever using yeast; remember that the yeast enzymes are still alive after the dough is baked. Place the baked dough in the refrigerator for three days.

Recipe 29 ——————————————

Coconut Oatmeal Carob Roma Cookies

Mix in a large bowl:

Four teaspoons of almond butter

Six cups of maple syrup

Two teaspoons of bio-salt

Three tablespoons of Roma

Three tablespoons of carob

8.8 ounces of coconut lite (a fine, dry, powdered coconut)

Four cups of oatmeal flour (Oatmeal flour is whole oats placed in a blender.)

Let sit for one to two hours, especially if dough is too moist. Bake for thirty minutes at 325 degrees. Place on trays using cookie mat or parchment paper. Place trays in oven one at a time.

Recipe 30 ——————————————

Coconut Oatmeal cookies

Place in a large bowl all the following and mix:

Four cups of oatmeal flour (Oatmeal flour is made by placing 100% whole oats in a blender.)

8.8 ounces of coconut lite (a powdered coconut)

Six cups of maple syrup

Two teaspoons of bio-salt

Four teaspoons of almond butter

Mix and let sit for one to two hours. Bake in 325-degree oven for thirty minutes.

Place on trays; use cookie mat or parchment paper.

Place trays in oven one at a time.

Recipe 31 ———————————————————

Carob Roma Coconut Oatmeal Whole-Wheat Pastry Flour Cookies

Mix the following in a large bowl:

Six cups of maple syrup

Two tablespoons of almond butter

One teaspoon of bio-salt

One half cup of carob

One half cup of roma

<u>Mix and add:</u>

8.8 Ounces of Coconut Lite (a dry, powered coconut)

<u>Mix and add:</u>

Four cups of oatmeal flour (Oatmeal flour is made by placing oatmeal in a blender.)

<u>Mix and add:</u>

Five cups of whole-wheat pastry flour

Bake at 325 degrees for twenty-five minutes.

Place on trays; use cookie mat or parchment paper.

This recipe makes 75 cookies.

Five trays are required, fifteen per tray. If batter is thin, let it sit for one to two hours to thicken.

Recipe 32

Coconut Oatmeal Whole-Wheat Pastry Flour Cookies

Mix the following in a bowl:

Two teaspoon of almond butter

Six cups of maple syrup

One teaspoon of bio-salt

8.8 ounces of Coconut Lite (a fine, dry, powdered coconut)

Four cups of oatmeal flour (Oatmeal flour is made by placing whole oatmeal in the blender.)

Five cups of whole-wheat pastry flour, sifted

Bake at 325 degrees for twenty-five minutes. Place on trays; use cookie mat or parchment paper. This recipe makes 75 cookies. Five trays are required, fifteen per tray.

If batter is thin, let it sit for one to two hours to thicken. Place trays one at a time in oven.

Recipe 33 ———————————————

Stuffed Bell Peppers

You will need: fourteen red, green, yellow, and orange bell peppers.

Cut a circle on the top of the bell peppers and remove the seeds. Save the top. Boil bell peppers in two cups of water, seven at a time, for 15 minutes. Use lid to cover pan while boiling. Let peppers cool.

In another pan, boil the following for 5-10 minutes:

One onion, cut small

Four tablespoons of Braggs-amino

One tablespoon of maple syrup

One can of green olives, each cut in half

One half cup of cilantro, cut small

One teaspoon of paprika

One teaspoon of bio-salt

One tablespoon of garlic powder

Three tablespoons of lemon juice

Two tablespoons of parsley

Continue to boil and stir

For the rice, do this the night before. In a large oven dish with lid place the following

One tablespoon bio-salt, ten cups of water and six cups of rice

The next day bake in oven at 250 degrees for two hours

Remove from oven and add rice to the above large pan and mix ingredients

Then spoon mixture into bell peppers

Replace bell pepper lid

In a glass dish bake at 325 degrees for thirty minutes

Recipe 34 ———————————————————————

Maple Syrup Cookies

Mix the following in a large bowl:

One teaspoon of vanilla

One teaspoon of bio-salt

One teaspoon of rosewater

One teaspoon of almond butter

Four cups of maple syrup

Six cups of ground walnuts

Four cups of whole-wheat pastry flour, sifted

This recipe makes 84 cookies; seven trays, and twelve per tray.

Use a baking mat or parchment paper; if dough is sticky, let sit for one to two hours. Bake in 325-degree oven for 25 minutes.

Recipe 35 ————————————————————

Carob Cookies

Mix the following in a large bowl:

One teaspoon of vanilla

One tablespoon of bio-salt

One tablespoon of rose water

Four cups of maple syrup

One tablespoon of almond butter

Four tablespoons of carob

Four tablespoons of Roma

Six cups of ground walnuts

Four cups of whole-wheat pastry flour sifted

Place on trays with cookie mat or parchment paper, and bake at 325 degrees for 25 minutes.

This recipe makes 84 cookies, and needs seven trays, twelve to each tray.

If dough is sticky, let it set for one to two hours.

Recipe 36 _____

Carob Brown Cake

Mix the following in a large bowl:

Three-quarter cup of soy milk

One-half teaspoon of bio-salt

One-third cup of maple syrup

One teaspoon of vanilla

One-third cup of sucanat sugar

One-half cup of carob

One tablespoon of roma

Two-thirds cup of whole-wheat pastry flour, sifted

Mix and place into a cake pan (9 x 9) lined with parchment paper and bake at 350 degrees for 25 minutes.

Check to see if the cake is done by placing a toothpick in the center of the cake. If nothing is on the toothpick once you've pulled it out, then the cake is done. If there is batter on the toothpick, leave the cake in the oven for another five minutes. You can place frosting on the top of the cake or enjoy as is.

Recipe Order List

57 ROBERT E MENZIE WALNUT PIE

58 APRICOT COCONUT WALNUT SQUARES

59 PISTACHIO SCONES

60 EGG ROLLS

61 ROASTED SALTED NUTS

62 FUDGE CUP COOKIE

63 FUDGE SAUCE

64 PINEAPPLE COOKIES

65 TAMALE BEAN PIE

66 NUT PIE

67 DATE-WALNUT COOKIES

68 CARAMELIZED GINGER HAZELNUT TART

69 PAPAYA COOKIES

70 CAJUN MIXED NUTS

71 TACO SALAD SHELLS

72 FOR CAKE-WEDDING STYLE CAKE

73 SPANISH MILLET CASSEROLE

74 ENCHILADAS

75 CAROB PIE

76 NUT BUTTER BALLS

77 SHARAREH SHABAFROOZ GARLIC BREAD SPREAD/BUTTER

78 GLAZED CARROT CAKE

79 WAFFLES WITH CASHEWS AND OATMEAL

80 LEMON PINEAPPLE PIE

81 CORN BREAD

82 MATTHEW F. MOONEY ROAST FOR ANY HOLIDAY

83 SPICE DOUGHNUTS

84 SPANISH RICE

85 PINEAPPLE SANDWICH COOKIE

86 CAROB CUP COOKIE

87 ANY FRUIT CUP COOKIE

88 SETAREH TAIS CAKE

89 CAROB DATE PISTACHIO PASTRY

90 FRUIT CAKE COOKIE

91 BAKED MILLET

92 BISCOTTI

93   MULTIGRAIN CRACKERS

94   POT PIE

95   BASIC COOKIE WITH FROSTING

96   TACO SHELLS

97   ANY FRUIT PASTRY

98   PINEAPPLE FROSTING

99   PINEAPPLE UPSIDE DOWN CAKE

100   HOT BEANS FOR BURRITOS

101   APRICOT PIE

102   APPLE PIE

103   PLUM PIE

104   PIZZA SAUCE NO. 3

105   PIZZA SAUCE NO. 1

106   COFFEE MUFFINS

107   GLORIA DUGGINS PECAN CANDY

108   PETER P. PANAGOPOULOS ALMOND FUDGE

109   PETE/ROSA CERRILLO CINNAMON WALNUT CANDY

110   SUGARED NUTS

111   PAPAYA CANDY

112   CAROB CAKE

113   THELMA MAIN HAZELNUT FUDGE

114   WHEAT CORNMEAL PIZZA

115   MARGARET/HARVEY BINDER PECAN FUDGE

116   MICHAEL F. MOONEY PECAN ROMA CAROB CANDY

117   BELLE HUCK WALNUT FUDGE

118   SAUCE FOR INSIDE CINNAMON ROLLS

119   NECTARINE PIE

120   COOKIES/CAROB PLAIN OR ROMA

121   CAROB BARS

122   SPICE BUTTER COOKIES

123   OAT CRACKERS

124   CINNAMON SUGAR DOUGHNUT TOPPING

125   JELLY DOUGHNUT FILLING

126   STRUDEL DOUGH

127   DATE CUP COOKIE

128   ITALIAN SAUCE

129 LASAGNA

130 BOB PANAGOPOULOS PIZZA SAUCE NO. 2

131 CUBAN BLACK BEANS IN RICE

132 BLACK BEANS

133 LIGHT FUDGE

134 DARK FUDGE

135 PIGEON BEANS

136 XENIA PANAGOPOULOS PIGEON RICE

137 ALEXANDRA PANAGOPOULOS SWEET AND SOUR SAUCE NO. 1

138 INEZ SPEIDELL SWEET AND SOUR SAUCE NO. 2

139 VERY VERY HOT SAUCE

140 LENTILS

141 SHRIMP SAUCE

142 GABRIEL CERRILLO ALMOND CAROB CANDY

143 CAROB ROMA CANDY

144 WALNUT CINNAMON CLUSTERS

145 TAMARA NEUMILLER SPANISH PASTA

146 CHINESE RICE

147 CHILI BEANS

148 TAMALES

149 VEGETABLE SOUP

150 CAROB ROMA COOKIES

151 RAY AND LINDA PANAGOPOULOS SUNFLOWER
      COCONUT WAFFLES

152 WAFFLES OATMEAL AND ALMONDS

153 RHI CAROB AND ROMA OATMEAL WWP NUTLESS COOKIE

154 HOT SAUCE

155 RED BEANS FOR TOP OF RICE

156 CORN MEAL WAFFLES

157 TAGLIATELLE SAUCE

158 ALMOND BUTTER COOKIES

159 MAPLE SYRUP FROSTING

160 ORANGE GLAZE

161 RYE PANCAKES

162 PANCAKES

163 BLUEBERRY TOPPING

199 MARSELLAS PANAGOPOULOS BRAZIL NUT ICE CREAM

200 TAHEREH MALEK PUMPKIN ICE CREAM

201 BAKED BROWN RICE

202 GINGER CANDY

203 SANDY MOONEY COFFEE CAKE

204 PAPAYA WALNUT COOKIES

205 LEMON CARROT COOKIES

206 CAROB SANDWICH COOKIES

207 DAISY FROSTING

208 BLACK-EYED PEAS

209 ALMOND BUTTER FROSTING

210 CRUNCH TOPPING FOR ANY BAKED PIE

211 CHERI GILBERT COOKED CAROB GLAZE

212 SUCANANT SUGAR GLAZE

213 ROMA CREAM FROSTING

214 LEMON FILLING

215 BAR-B-QUE SAUCE

216 TOFU FROSTING

217 SWEET SUGAR ICING

218 BLACK EYED IN RICE

219 SOY MILK CORNBREAD

220 OATMEAL ALMOND COOKIE

221 SPICED CUPCAKES

222 DATE OATMEAL COOKIE

223 ORANGE COCONUT COOKIE

224 DATE COOKIE BAR

225 APRICOT COOKIE BAR

226 GINGER PANCAKES

227 LEMON PASTRY

228 LEMON SUGAR COOKIES

229 DATE BROWNIES

230 ORIGINAL SALT WATER TAFFY

231 AURA VICTORIA HUCK PEPPERMINT SALT WATER TAFFY

232 LEMON SALT WATER TAFFY

233 VANILLA SALT WATER TAFFY

234 ORANGE SALT WATER TAFFY

235 JACK PANAGOPOULOS ROMA SALT WATER TAFFY
236 ADRIANA CERRILLO PECAN SALT WATER TAFFY
237 ELMER LYLE MENZIE ALMOND SALT WATER TAFFY
238 ASHLEY SPEIDELL WALNUT SALT WATER TAFFY
239 ROSS H. MENZIE CAROB SALT WATER TAFFY
240 COCONUT SALT WATER TAFFY
241 CINAMMON SALT WATER TAFFY
242 GINGER SALT WATER TAFFY
243 GENE KOENING ENGLISH TOFFEE CANDY
244 LUCILLE GILBERT LEMON CHEESECAKE
245 ORANGE CHEESECAKE
246 ASHER MICHAEL NEUMILLER CAROB CHEESECAKE
247 ALLIE NICOLE BLUMA NEUMILLER CAROB CAKE
248 DR. EDE VANILLA SUGAR CAKE
249 WALNUT SQUARE COOKIES
250 TARA SHABAFROOZ PECAN SQUARE COOKIES
251 ALMOND SQUARE COOKIES
252 MARGRET ANN MENZIE PECAN ROPE COOKIES
253 MASSOOD SHABAFROOZ WALNUT ROPE COOKIES
254 ALMOND ROPE COOKIES

14 Days of Meals

The purpose of this fourteen-day meal plan is to illustrate that starvation does not exist when following the plan. Instead of listing the fruit on a daily log every day, I just list here approximately what was eaten. For the last two years, I have reversed my two meals. The larger was consumed first and the second is mostly raw. Prior to eating breakfast, generally a half an hour after I wake, I drink a quart of warm water with two teaspoons of lemon juice, one tablespoon of Inland sea water, and one tablespoon of silver mineral water.

I consume approximately five pounds of fruit daily, and the fruit varies according to the seasons of the year.

These fourteen days are very similar (fruit meal) and they are: three different colors of apples, twelve cherries, one nectarine, one mango, one slice of pineapple, one slice of cantaloupe, eight green grapes, one apricot, and one peach. In addition, I also eat eight raw Brazil nuts, six apricot nuts, one teaspoon of sunflower seeds, one teaspoon of pumpkin seeds, two capsules of calcium, and two capsules of magnesium.

For dinner, I usually have a salad which consists of:

Red head lettuce

Three radishes cut small

One long green onion, cut small

One third of a carrot, cut small

Half of an avocado

Half of celery stalk, cut small

Six tablespoons of lemon juice

Approximately one tablespoon of Braggs-amino

Up to twelve ounces or more of two different kinds of hot sauce

Bread, crackers, or corn tortillas

Day #1   **Breakfast:** Fruit and a sunflower-seed waffle.

Dinner: Salad, one quarter pound of crackers, two egg rolls, twelve ounces of Chinese rice.

Dessert: One quarter pound of walnut fudge.

Day #2   **Breakfast:** Fruit and six ounces of Cajun rice with Braggs-amino and lemon juice.

Dinner: Salad, four baked potatoes, six corn tortillas, twelve ounces of Texan rice.

Dessert: One quarter pound of cinnamon roll.

Day #3   **Breakfasts:** Fruit and bowl of oatmeal.

Dinner: Salad, twelve ounces of pan-fried noodles, twelve ounces of Chinese rice, and one serving of a quarter pound of bread.

Dessert: One quarter pound of pineapple pie.

Day #4   **Breakfast:** Fruit and one slice of toast with apricot jam for toast.

Dinner: Salad, twelve ounces of plain brown rice, twelve ounces of lentils, one quarter pound of bread.

Dessert: One quarter pound of peach turnovers.

Day #5   **Breakfasts:** Fruit, oatmeal waffle.

Dinner: Salad, one quarter pound of crackers, 24 ounces of vegetable soup.

Dessert: One quarter pound pecan candy bars.

Day #6   **Breakfasts:** Fruit, six ounces of Cajun nut mix.

Dinner: Salad, one quarter pound of bread, one and one half pounds of pasta, including twelve ounces of tomato sauce.

Dessert: One quarter pound Robert E Menzie Walnut pie

Day # 7   **Breakfast:** Fruit, large bowl of popcorn sprayed with Braggs-amino.

Dinner: Salad, two stuffed bell peppers, one quarter pound of crackers, twelve ounces of rice.

Dessert: One quarter pound of pecan fudge.

Day #8   **Breakfasts:** Fruit and one slice of toast with cherry jam.

Dinner: Salad, one pot pie, one quarter pound of crackers, six ounces of Puerto Rican Rice, with the pot pie.

Dessert: One quarter pound of lemon ice cream.

Day #9   **Breakfasts:** Fruit, cornmeal waffle.

Dinner: Salad, two bean burritos, twelve ounces of Spanish rice, and six Corn tortillas.

Dessert: One quarter pound of pineapple cookies.

Day #10   **Breakfasts:** Fruit, one pancake.

Dinner: Salad, one and one half pounds of Spanish lasagna, one quarter pound of crackers.

Dessert: One quarter pound of carob coconut cookies.

Day #11   **Breakfast:** Fruit, one bowl oatmeal.

Dinner: Salad, pizza, one quarter pound crackers.

Dessert: One quarter pound of golden macaroon cookies.

Day #12   **Breakfasts:** Fruit, six ounces of Puerto Rican rice, with lemon juice and Braggs-amino.

Dinner: Salad, one pound of tamale bean pie, six ounces Spanish rice, one quarter pound bread.

Dessert: One quarter pound of carob pie.

Day #13   **Breakfasts:** Fruit, one slice of toast with almond butter.

Dinner: Open-face sandwiches, four slices of toast, two plates of salad on top of the toast. Add twelve ounces of hot sauce, three spoons of lemon juice, and sprinkle with Braggs-amino on top for taste.

Dessert: One quarter pound of baked Alaska.

Day #14   **Breakfasts:** Fruit, six ounces of Texan rice.

Dinner: Salad, one-quarter pound of crackers, 24 ounces of Chinese soup.

Dessert: One quarter pound carob cake.

Conclusion

Eating unhealthily will only cost you more, for imitation nutrition, and will cause a loss of a good life.

This is the cause of being overweight, not the lack of drugs, or starvation diets. So how can it be the solution? As you know by now, this book is not just another new diet plan; instead, it is a plan of weight loss according to your body's ideal weight, including basic cooking, setting up your pantry, and cooking tips. These are real doable solutions. New abilities and possibilities will be obvious. The impossible will be possible. Happiness, higher quality of life, and a new beginning will occur. Limitation will be eliminated. All this has happened to me and more. This is yours if you want, and do not be surprised if you notice other changes in your body. Within eight to twenty-six days, there will be major changes in your weight loss. This weight loss will stay off if improper nutrition is not part of your daily life. Instead of treating your body like garbage can, care for it, because it is priceless.

It is very important to do what works and quit listening to anyone who promotes methods that do not work! Education or knowledge is everywhere and not limited to a college or university. I have done thousands of hours of independent research, and this will continue. It is really common sense that everyone will make improvements in their daily life, to restore and achieve radiant health.

Please do not copy or give away any material, not just because it is copyright-protected material, but doing this will interfere with my program of feeding and educating the unhealthy. Instead, my wish is that you do share your cooking with friends, family, and strangers.

Questions, concerns and suggestions are welcomed.

24-hour message phone: 559-435-4069

This line will also have some general information, updates, Web sites, information, and new recipes. The price of recipes is to be announced on the Web site.

Want a recipe named after you or a friend? The cost is $2,600.

Want an autographed book? Price is to be announced on Web site.

To order or inquire about the Cellerciser™

Call 1-800-856-4863.

For a substantial discount, mention my name.

Send written comments to:

Frederick M. Huck

P.O. Box 27911

Fresno, CA 93729-7911

Please visit us at www.frederickhuck.com.

References

Dr. Ede Koenig, Founder and President of Radiant Health Institute and School of Radiant Health, D.S.C., Ph.D., N.M.D.N.D

Author of *the Whole Kernel*
See the Dangers if any Oil in the Body

Dr. Wendell Stanley, eminent virus scientist, Nobel Prize 1957,

Written over 150 papers, Nobel lecture, and Chemistry 1942-1962

Elsevier Publishing Co., Amsterdam 1964

See the Dangers of Eating Animal Products

Dr. Otto Warburg won the Nobel Prize in Medicine in 1931 and 1944.

Foreign Member of the Royal Society of London, a Knight of the Order of Merit

And honorary degrees from Harvard, Oxford, and Heidelberg.

See the 1966 Annual Meeting of the Novelists at Lindau, Germany.

See the Dangers of Sugar in the Human Body

About the Author

Frederick Mickel Huck is an advocate and promoter of good, healthy eating, being involved in years of independent research in health-related articles, videos, seminars, and testimonials. He strives for variety in food preparation with building upon recipe information through countless cooking experiments. He has shared his cooking secrets through teaching basic cooking sessions on updated sanitary cooking methods, proper cooking utensils, food storage, and notes on product selection and availability.

Frederick has also entered local cooking contests and contributed many hours of sponsoring food samples to interested audiences. He has given away more than one hundred thousand personally baked cookies and other foods. He believes that by replacing all junk food with healthy food, which looks and tastes better, your body will function and age better with nurturing nutrients.

Frederick has lost fifty-five pounds within two months after discovering and making the changes in his food selection and preparation. He attributes his good health and well-being to minor workout and eating balance and properly prepared meals. He had problems with diabetes, kidney stones, and bone problems, which were virtually eliminated with his daily commitment of striving for a good, healthy body. He states that his body feels clean and that his mind seems to be more alert and sharper.

www.ingramcontent.com/pod-product-compliance
Lightning Source LLC
Chambersburg PA
CBHW052011280526
45793CB00005B/934